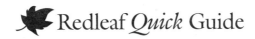

Redleaf *Quick* Guide

Recognizing Common Illnesses

IN EARLY CHILDHOOD SETTINGS

Hilary Pert Stecklein, MD

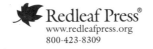

Redleaf Press®
www.redleafpress.org
800-423-8309

Published by Redleaf Press
10 Yorkton Court
St. Paul, MN 55117
www.redleafpress.org

First edition 2010 by Redleaf Press
Interior typeset in Univers
Interior illustration by Elizabeth Bub
Printed in the United States of America
16 15 14 13 12 11 10 09   1 2 3 4 5 6 7 8

Library of Congress Cataloging-in-Publication Data
Stecklein, Hilary Pert.
  Recognizing common illnesses in early childhood settings / Hilary Pert Stecklein. — 1st ed.
     p. cm. — (Redleaf quick guide)
  ISBN 978-1-933653-67-9
  1. Children—Diseases—Handbooks, manuals, etc. 2. Symptoms in children—Handbooks, manuals, etc.
3. School health services—Handbooks, manuals, etc. 4. Early childhood education—Handbooks, manuals,
etc. I. Title.
  RJ48.S74 2009
  618.92—dc22
                                        2009004845
Printed on acid-free paper

Recognizing Common Illnesses in Early Childhood Settings

Introduction

Hilary Pert Stecklein, MD

Welcome! This book provides a first aid guide to what you need to know about common illnesses in children. It will teach you

- how to recognize illness;

- how to recognize when an illness or symptom may be dangerous;

- how to take care of the ill child and protect the others in your care;

- how to prevent problems.

Remember: it is never up to you to diagnose an illness. But the families of children in your care are counting on you to know what to do when a child is ill. They will look to you to make your nurturing child care setting as comforting and safe as possible.

How This Book Is Organized

This book begins by explaining why children are at risk for germs, provides information about germ patterns, and describes how you can tell that a child is ill. It provides specific answers to the following questions about each of the illnesses common in early childhood settings:

- Is this an emergency?

- What germs can cause this problem?

- What is the likely pattern of this illness?

- How is this germ spread?

- How much time elapses between being infected and becoming ill?

- When can the child spread the germ?

- What are the possible complications?

- Can you be immune?

- What comfort care may be needed?

- How can you keep the germs from being spread?

- How long should the ill child be kept out of child care?

- What treatments may be needed once the child returns?

It also includes information about vaccines, guidelines for cleanliness, and a list of helpful resources.

Hilary Pert Stecklein, MD, is a pediatrician with twenty-two years of clinical experience. Trained at Wellesley College, the State University of New York, the University of South Florida, and Harvard Medical School's Children's Hospital Boston, Dr. Stecklein is a clinical associate professor in pediatrics at the University of Minnesota and former CEO of the medical office-based family reading program, Reading Rx. She practices pediatrics and adolescent medicine at HealthPartners in Saint Paul, Minnesota. She has won many community awards, including the Children's Hospitals and Clinics of Minnesota's Blanton Bessinger Child Advocacy Award. She is a frequently requested speaker and enjoys teaching medical information in ways that make sense and are useful to nonmedical people. Her interests include family literacy, family interaction, maximizing human development, medical education, and violence prevention.

Part 1: General Information about Germs

Kids Are At Great Risk for Catching Germs

Children in child care are at risk for catching certain infectious illnesses. Infections come from many kinds of germs—viruses, bacteria, parasites, and fungi. Whether being exposed to a certain germ makes a child sick or not depends on several things, including

- the type of germ and its infectiousness;

- the route and amount of contamination;

- individual immunity and ability to fight infection.

The best way to keep children healthy in child care is to have a clear plan that minimizes the risk of infection and maximizes possible protection. Controlling infection in early childhood settings requires action from families, children, and staff.

Key Factors Putting Children at Risk for Infection

1. **Cleanliness:** Personal hygiene really makes the biggest difference.

2. **Germ risk from the staff:** The health and immunization status of each child care provider have great impact on the overall risk of infection.

3. **Susceptibility of the children**: The age, immunization status, and health of each child in the program affect how susceptible to infection he or she will be.

4. **Additional risk of exposure**: Outside of the child care setting, children come in contact with other sources of infection. For example, a child may have older siblings who are exposed to an infection at school.

5. **Ratio of children to care provider:** The number of children per provider affects the overall risk for illness. The risk increases with a greater number of children per provider.

6. **Physical environment:** The physical setup of the child care setting plays a role in health because it affects how easy or hard the environment is to keep clean and sanitary. For example, the number of sinks and their location affect how easy it is for everyone to wash their hands regularly.

7. **Training and practice:** A well-trained staff that follows established health procedures plays an important role in preventing the spread of illness. The choice of and frequency of cleaning materials also make a huge difference.

> Hand washing by families, children, and child care staff is the most important and effective prevention of all.

1

Special Factors Putting Infants and Toddlers At Risk for Infection

Some developmental-stage behaviors make it more likely for infants and toddlers to catch and share germs.

- Infants and toddlers need direct help with feeding.

- Infants and toddlers need direct help with diaper and toilet care.

- Young children do not control their body fluids well, including saliva and spit, nasal drainage, coughs, sneezes, vomit, urine, and stool.

- Young children have had little time to develop immunity to common germs.

- Young children explore their world not just through seeing and hearing but also by smelling, tasting, and touching with eager fingers and mouths. These explorations include touching other children.

- Young children are less likely to understand boundaries and rules.

- Young children haven't developed healthy hygiene habits yet.

What Makes a Germ Likely to Spread?

Each germ has its own special pattern of hosts, incubation period between catching the germ and actually becoming sick, and infectiousness—the period during which a sick person can spread the germ to other people. Some germs can be spread before the infected person shows any signs of illness. Each germ also can remain contagious in the environment for a particular time.

As a child care provider, you need to know how likely a particular germ is to be present in your program, how it can spread, and how to best to control its spread. Your germ management must be consistent and effective to protect uninfected children and staff.

Some germs spread easily, such as the varicella-zoster virus (which causes chicken pox) and the respiratory syncytial virus (or RSV, which causes severe respiratory diseases such as bronchiolitis). Others are very difficult to spread, like the human immunodeficiency virus (HIV) or the Epstein-Barr virus (which causes mononucleosis or mono).

> When children are contagious, they can spread the germs throughout the child care group, back to their homes, and out to the larger community.

How Do Germs Spread?

Some germs are spread in only one way, while others are spread in a variety of ways. The most common methods are

- Droplets in the air and on surfaces

- Stool and urine

- Saliva, spit, and drool

- Blood

- Skin

DROPLETS IN THE AIR AND ON SURFACES

You have probably seen pictures of the droplets that are emitted when someone sneezes or coughs. A sneeze or cough produces droplets that, depending on their size, can settle on surfaces, remain suspended in the air, or travel remarkable distances. Germs in these droplets may spread by being breathed in or absorbed into the body through the membranes of the nose, mouth, eyes, or sometimes skin; they may also be ingested. Droplets that land on or are wiped onto toys, hands, and doorknobs can spread and contaminate all surfaces and objects. The tiniest droplets often travel the farthest. Such germs include chicken pox (a virus that causes a classic skin rash but that also can cause brain infections and pneumonia) and measles (a virus that causes a different classic rash and that can produce many serious complications, including joint problems and brain infections). Larger droplets fall sooner and so typically spread over shorter distances. They also can be breathed in and spread by contact when they settle. Examples in this group include the common cold (caused by several different kinds of viruses), whooping cough (caused by *Bordetella pertussis*, a bacterium that can also cause pneumonia), and fifth disease (also called slapped face disease, caused by the parvovirus, which produces rash, fever, mouth and throat sores, and other symptoms).

STOOL

Even the smallest amounts of stool containing germs can make other people sick. Microscopic germs can be spread from a contaminated hand to another person's mouth directly or through contaminated toys and other objects or surfaces. These stool germs can also be spread through contaminated food or water. Germs that travel this way include giardia (a parasite), thrush (a yeast fungus), rotovirus (a virus that causes severe diarrhea, which can lead quickly to dehydration), the virus hepatitis A, which causes jaundice and liver problems, and *Salmonella* (a bacteria that can cause bloody diarrhea).

URINE

Urine only rarely carries germs that can be spread, but when an infectious agent is found in urine, it can be transferred from soiled hands or indirectly through surface contamination to someone else's mouth. An example is cytomegalovirus, which can cause many problems, including liver problems.

SALIVA, SPIT, AND DROOL

Germs from spit, saliva, and drool can spread by direct contact, including bites, or by contact with objects children use. Infants and toddlers who suck on or chew materials, including toys that are merely touched or shared, are at heightened risk. Examples of infections that can spread through saliva, spit, and drool include cytomegalovirus and Epstein-Barr (EBV), the virus that causes mononucleosis, which may produce sore throat and liver and spleen problems.

BLOOD

Some germs can be spread when infected blood comes into direct contact with another person's broken skin or mucous membranes. Some germs can be spread indirectly when germs from blood-contaminated objects are introduced into another person's circulatory system through broken skin or mucous membranes. This can happen even if the quantity of blood is too small to be visible. Some germs are infectious even when they have dried. Examples of germs spread from blood include the hepatitis B virus, which causes liver problems, and the hepatitis C virus, which also attacks the liver and more.

SKIN

Some germs are spread when secretions from an infected person come into contact with another person's soft, moist membranes. These special membranes are found not only in the nose but also in the eyes, mouth, and parts of the abdomen and genitals. These germs can be spread directly, through person-to-person contact, or indirectly, through contaminated objects and surfaces. They can enter through broken skin from cuts, scrapes, or sores. Examples of germs that spread through skin-to-skin contact include the virus that causes molluscum contagiosum (a wart), ringworm (a fungus that causes sores, including on the scalp), staphylococcus or streptococcus, bacteria that cause impetigo, and the viruses and bacteria that cause pink eye.

Recognizing a Child Who Is Ill (ɪll)

You know the children in your care. Changes in how they look, how they act, or how they feel may be the first signs of illness. Watch for these signs, and trust your instincts.

- Changes in breathing, including faster breathing

- Severe, deep or ongoing coughing

- Headache and/or stiff neck

- Less appetite or loss of appetite

- Fever or flushed body or face

- Rashes or other skin changes, including lumps or bumps

- Yellow eyes or skin

- Pus, redness, swelling, or other changes to the eye

- Vomiting

- Loose stool or diarrhea

- Sore throat or difficulty eating or swallowing

- Odd color or smell to urine

- Discomfort, fussy or cranky behavior

- Unusual activity, less or more than usual

What to Do When You Suspect a Child Is Ill

1. Evaluate whether or not the situation is an emergency.

2. Once you are sure the child is stable and the illness is not an emergency, separate the child from the other children.

3. Make sure all other child care staff know what is going on.

4. Contact the child's family or guardian.

5. Arrange for the child to go home as soon as possible.

Excluding a Child or Staff Member Who Is Ill

Child care is critical for many families. When that care is interrupted by the illness of a child or a care provider, the family can become very stressed. You can help these families by providing clear rules about when an ill person—a staff member or a child—must be kept out of the child care setting. Exclusion depends on many factors: the time a person is infectious, the likelihood of spreading germs, and the level of hygiene and other care needed and possible. Families need clearly stated policies about what accommodations can be made—if any—for a sick child. They need to understand that your center must minimize the risk of spreading infection to other children or staff on site while offering ill children comfort, safety, and solicitude until they can be sent home. Clearly written policies help families by setting realistic expectations for everyone.

Each illness has its own pattern of infectiousness and symptoms. (Please refer to specific illnesses in part 2 for more details.) It is very important to provide parents and staff with an illness policy that explains what symptoms exclude a staff member or a child from your program.

Here are some symptoms to include when you are setting your policy for excluding those who are ill:

- Fever equal to or higher than 100.5 F
- Significant amounts of clear or colored drainage from mouth, nose, ears, or eyes
- Redness of the white of the eyes or yellow discharge from the eyes
- Body rashes with fever
- Abdominal pain, vomiting, or diarrhea
- Painful red throat
- Deep cough, difficulty breathing, or wheezing
- Headache or stiff neck
- Yellow color to the skin or in the white of the eye
- Open sores or cuts that ooze, contain pus, or are very red or tender

Part 2: Recognizing Common Childhood Illnesses

Symptoms and Signs

The families of children in your care are counting on you to know what to do when a child is ill. And they will look to you to make your child care setting as comforting and safe as possible.

This book is organized by the main symptoms that children may exhibit. Almost every illness involves more than one part of the body and includes fever, vague aches, and/or a generalized feeling of not being well. Symptoms (what children feel and you can observe) and signs (what you can see) may vary and overlap from one germ pattern to another. This book draws on an approach that nurses and medical doctors use: identifying the main presenting problem. The main presenting problem is the primary thing the patient complains about or the signs someone else observes.

Many germs cause the same symptoms and signs, yet are very different in terms of the risks they pose to people. The symptom a child is most likely to experience and you to notice first is what this book describes, which will help you organize your approach. And as always, trust your instincts.

> Remember: it is never up to you to diagnose an illness.

What Are the Most Common Illnesses?

The most common illnesses covered in this book fall into nine general categories.

1. Shock and anaphylactic allergic reaction

2. Airway and breathing problems

3. Sore throat

4. Abdominal and digestive problems

5. Inflamed eyes

6. Joint problems

7. Rashes and other skin or scalp changes

8. Urinary tract infections

9. Ear infections

Shock and Anaphylactic Allergic Reaction

IS THIS AN EMERGENCY?

Shock is total body failure. It is always an emergency. Anaphylaxis is also always an emergency.

Call 911 immediately if you ever believe the child has an emergency situation.

Keep the child protected.

Inform the family or guardian immediately.

Refer to the *Medical Emergencies in Early Childhood Settings* Redleaf Quick Guide or another first aid manual as needed.

Shock has many causes, including

- bleeding;

- dehydration;

- severe airway, heart, or kidney disease;

- severe poisons;

- many kinds of infections and severe allergic reactions.

The most severe form of allergic response is called *anaphylaxis* or *anaphylactic reaction*. This can be caused by an immune response to

- foods;

- medications;

- insect bites.

For more information about allergic reactions, including food allergies, see the *Medical Emergencies in Early Childhood Settings* Redleaf Quick Guide.

The most severe kinds of infections that cause shock are caused by bacteria that infect the blood stream (bacteremia). Others include brain infections (meningitis and encephalitis), respiratory infections (pneumonia), and kidney infections (pyelonephritis).

What germs can cause this problem?

Infections that enter the blood stream (bacteremia) cause blood poisoning. When the infection overwhelms the body's defenses, it is called *sepsis*. A downward spiral of effects can lead to shock, collapse, and, in some cases, death.

The most common germs causing shock for children are members of the genus Staphylococcus. *Streptococcus pneumoniae*, *Haemophilus influenza* type b, and *Pseudomonas aeruginosa* are other important bacteria that can cause sepsis. *Neisseria meningitidis* can cause meningitis and over-whelming sepsis in adolescents and young adults. *Herpes simplex* virus, *Listeria monocytogenes*, and Group B streptococcus are risks for newborns in particular. Infants and children who are seri-ously injured or have other chronic medical problems are at greatest risk. The immunization of infants against *H. influenza* type b and *Strep pneumoniae* and of teenagers for *Neisseria meningitidis* has dramatically decreased these kinds of infections. (See the section on immunization on page 45.)

What is the likely pattern of this illness?

Anaphylaxis can show as paleness or blue-color changes in the lips, face, gums, and fingers. Children may have generalized hives or itch-flush skin rash. They may have swollen lips, tongue, and uvula. They may have cold and clammy skin, agitation, or sleepiness. Breathing problems, including breath-ing fast; noisy breathing, including stridor (a high-pitched breathing sound); or wheezing may occur. They can have abdominal pain (cramps) and vomiting or gagging. Ill children may have either high or low temperatures, fast or slow heartbeats, abnormally low blood pressure.

How is this germ spread?

The germs that can ultimately cause shock from sepsis are usually spread through the airway. These germs can be directly spread by droplet (through cough or sneeze) or indirectly spread through fresh contamination by an infected person's hands on toys, surfaces, and utensils, including anything that may have been in contact with a contagious child's mouth, nose, or airway secretions, such as straws, silverware, and cups.

How much time elapses between being infected and becoming ill?

It depends on the germ, but it can be within a few hours.

When can the child spread the germ?

Some of these germs are extremely contagious, starting twenty-four to forty-eight hours before a child shows signs of illness. During this time, all direct contact is risky. Possible sepsis always requires medi-cal care. Because some of the germs can be extremely contagious and dangerous, it is important to get information and guidance from medical providers to determine if staff and other children are at risk.

What are the possible complications?

Blood clots, tissue abscesses, seizures, hemorrhages, delirium, multiple organ failure, coma, and even death.

Can you be immune?

Vaccination protects against many of these germs, especially *Streptococcus pneumoniae*, *Haemophilus influenzae* type b, and *Neisseria meningitidis*.

What comfort care may be needed?

Follow your emergency plan. Keep the child comfortable and protected. Isolate her from the other children, and minimize contact with other staff.

How can you keep the germs from being spread?

Be sure the child and all caregivers receive appropriate immunizations. Excellent hygiene, including aid with covering all coughs and sneezes with disposable tissue, teaching children to use their sleeves or elbows, and careful hand washing and cleaning of any contaminated surfaces or materials, is necessary to prevent transmission.

How long should the ill child be kept out of child care?

Until she has recovered and been cleared to return by her medical provider. The child should be feeling well, registering no fever, taking appropriate antibiotics, and otherwise doing well.

What treatments may be needed once the child returns?

The child will need to comply with any continuing medical care plan outlined by her medical provider.

Airway and Breathing Problems

IS THIS AN EMERGENCY?

Call 911 immediately if you ever believe the child has an emergency situation.

Keep the child protected.

Inform the family or guardian as soon as possible.

Refer to the *Medical Emergencies in Early Childhood Settings* Redleaf Quick Guide or another first aid manual as needed.

Oxygen is critical for survival; when it becomes unavailable, the child is endangered. This constitutes an emergency. If you are concerned about the child's breathing, look for these signs:

- Looks air-hungry

- Shows anxiety about breathing

- Pants or seems to have trouble breathing or moving air in or out

- Displays effortful breathing: skin is sucked in between the ribs or at the top of the chest in the notch above the breastplate or above the clavicle

- Changes colors, including red, pale and/or dusky, or blue around the mouth, the face, or elsewhere

- Makes a noise that sounds as if it is difficult to move air, including stridor (a high-pitched breathing sound) or harsh coughing

- Has trouble swallowing (includes drooling)

- Has difficulty catching the breath

SPECIAL NOTE about asthma

Asthma is the most common chronic disease of childhood, affecting more than six million children in the United States alone (National Center for Health Statistics). It is not an infection but rather the result of changes in the airways and tissues of the lungs. Asthma swells the lining of the airway and produces extra mucus and muscle spasms in the airway. Coughing and wheezing are the most common symptoms of childhood asthma. There are several patterns of asthma, including sudden attacks, which can be life threatening. **Remember: any problems with a child's breathing constitutes an emergency, and you need to follow emergency guidelines, including calling 911.** Children with asthma are particularly susceptible to airway infections and are more likely to become sick more quickly, more deeply, and for longer times because illnesses activate their asthma. Possible triggers include viral upper airway infections (especially those caused by RSV and rhinoviruses). Occasional nonviral infections, such as those caused by *Mycoplasma pneumoniae* and *Chlamydia trachomatis,* can be triggers as well. Allergies, exercise, weather changes, and tobacco smoke can trigger asthma. Children with asthma who are in your care need to have appropriate asthma care, including an "asthma action plan" from their family and medical provider that outlines the treatment plan for the child during child care.

Bacteria and Viruses

Most airway and breathing-problem infections are caused by either bacteria or viruses.

The most common bacterial infections are caused by *Streptococcus pneumoniae* (different from strep throat), *Haemophilus influenzae* type b (different from influenza), and *Bordetella pertussis* (whooping cough). *Mycobacterium tuberculosis* is a special kind of germ most like a bacterial germ. A rare but extremely dangerous infection is *Neisseria meningitidis.*

Airway and breathing viruses include those that cause common colds, influenza, RSV, and parainfluenza.

General Symptoms and Typical Patterns

Remember: asthma may produce a combination of symptoms, and you must always look at the whole child. Nevertheless, some typical patterns exist, and these primarily involve the main area of the airway. Breathing and the airway start at the nose and mouth and go through the throat, including the pharynx (back of the throat and nose), larynx (voice box in the upper throat), trachea (middle part of the airway in the neck, going down into the chest), bronchi (the main tubes that split into each side of the chest), bronchioles (the smaller branches of the breathing tree, deep in the chest), and end in the alveoli (the air sacks in the deepest part of lung tissue in which oxygen is exchanged).

The following illnesses are discussed in this chapter:

- Upper respiratory infections (common cold)
- Laryngeotracheobronchitis (LTB)/croup
- Bronchitis
- Bronchiolitis
- Pneumonia

Diagram of Child's Respiratory System

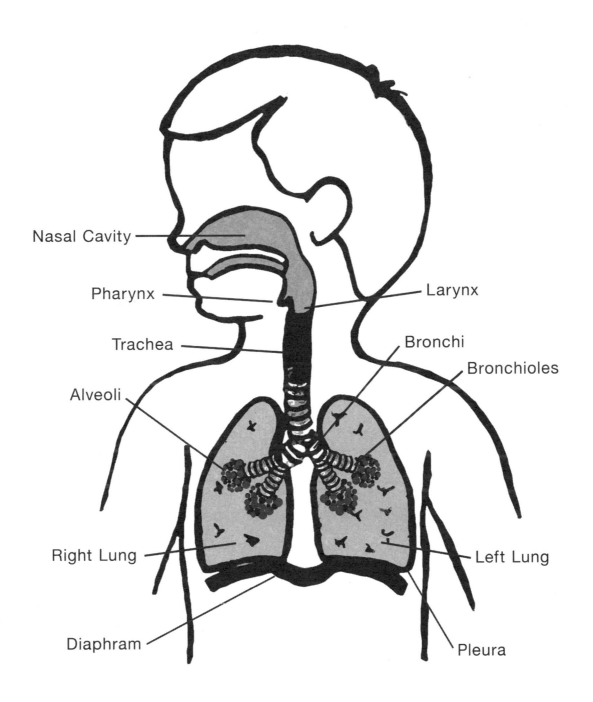

Nasal Cavity

Pharynx

Trachea

Alveoli

Right Lung

Diaphram

Larynx

Bronchi

Bronchioles

Left Lung

Pleura

Upper Respiratory Infections

Upper respiratory infections (URI) are typically known as common colds. These illnesses are very contagious and spread quickly. Signs include initial nasal secretions, congestion, nose tissue swelling, sneezing, mild sore throat, and low-grade fever.

How is this germ spread?
Cold germs are spread through the airway. These germs can be directly spread by droplet (through cough or sneeze) or indirectly spread through fresh contamination by an ill person's hands on toys, surfaces, and utensils, including anything that may have come into contact with a contagious child's mouth, nose, or airway secretions, such as straws, silverware, and cups.

How much time elapses between being infected and becoming ill?
One to three days.

When can the child spread the germ?
Starting a day or two before the child becomes ill, lasting at least seven to ten days.

What are the possible complications?
These viruses can cause many symptoms, including head congestion, sinus and ear pressure, and pain. Secondary infections, including bacterial infections, often develop in the mucus. These can become sinus and middle ear infections. Because most common colds take seven to ten days to complete, nasal drainage may go from clear to cloudy to yellow to green. If nasal drainage is consistently green for longer than seven to ten days, or if the child continues to experience high fevers or pain, he may need to see a medical provider for further evaluation.

 SPECIAL NOTE about ear infections

An ear infection is not directly contagious. The cold that sets the child up for an ear infection is what is contagious. By the time a child develops an ear infection, the cold is passing or has past. He should not be considered infectious and does not need to be restricted from child care if his comfort level and ability to handle normal activities are good.

 SPECIAL NOTE about sinusitis

Sinusitis is different from a common cold because it involves the air passages and deeper chambers within the head. These are lined with the same kind of tissue as the nose. Viral upper respiratory infections can cause inflammation of these chamber linings; they are common and usually resolve in thirty days or fewer. These linings can become superinfected by bacteria, but they rarely need evaluation and treatment. Chronic inflammation lasts more than thirty days with persistent symptoms, including cough, runny nose, and signs of blocked-up nose. It can be related to problems not connected to infection, including allergies, reflux (heartburn), smoke exposure, and other environmental pollutants. It should be evaluated.

Can you be immune?
You can be immune to an individual cold germ, but there are so many variations of these kinds of germs that most people continue to get new colds.

What comfort care may be needed?
Gentle nose skin care, extra humidity, and nasal saline may be given if directed by families. Please note: decongestants and antihistamines (cough and cold medicines) are not helpful and are potentially harmful for children; they are not recommended.

How can you keep the germs from being spread?
Excellent airway hygiene, including aid with covering all coughs and sneezes with disposable tissue, teaching children to use their sleeves or elbows, and careful hand washing and cleaning of any contaminated surfaces or materials, is necessary to prevent transmission.

How long should the ill child be kept out of child care?
It is not necessary to exclude a child with a mild cold who is comfortable and otherwise doing well, provided the hygiene necessary to control the infection is possible.

What treatments may be needed once the child returns?
Good hygiene is necessary to control the germs—hand washing and keeping possibly infected surfaces clean are critical.

Laryngeotracheobronchitis (LTB)/Croup

Also called *croup*, LTB is the inflammation and infection of the voice box and the uppermost section of the trachea (breathing tube).

What germs can cause this problem?
Laryngeotracheobronchitis is typically caused by viruses (RSV, adenovirus, influenza and parainfluenza viruses). It is rarely caused by bacteria, but an initial infection with mycoplasma can lead to LTB.

What is the likely pattern of this illness?
The child has initial cold symptoms that proceed to a hoarse voice and a classic, harsh barky cough (a hollow sound like that of a dog, seal, or goose). The cough tends to be worse at night. The child may also have sneezing, mild sore throat, and low-grade fever. The illness is rare after six years of age but can occur in children as young as three months. A second cycle of infection after the initial viral infection can occur with new germs, including *Streptococcus pneumoniae*, *Staphylococcus aureus*, and

others. Some children have a tendency to develop LTB with multiple infections and may have some underlying airway narrowing; they should be evaluated.

 SPECIAL NOTE about epiglotitis

A few special problems that are *not* LTB can start with very much the same symptoms. **Remember: any concern about a child's breathing is an emergency, and you need to follow emergency guidelines, including calling 911.** Epiglotitis, typically caused by *Haemophilus influenzae* type b, is an infection of the epiglottis (special airway flap) that separates the trachea (airway tube) from the esophagus (food tube). It can be extremely dangerous. Infected children usually show drooling and may experience rapidly progressive airway swelling that is life threatening.

How is this germ spread?
These germs can be directly spread by droplet (through cough or sneeze) or indirectly spread through fresh contamination by an ill person's hands on toys, surfaces, and utensils, including anything that may have been in contact with a contagious child's mouth, nose, or airway secretions, such as straws, silverware, and cups.

How much time elapses between being infected and becoming ill?
Typically two to five days.

When can the child spread the germ?
From the day the child is infected until at least three to five days after symptoms appear.

What are the possible complications?
Laryngeotracheobronchitis is rarely associated with secondary bacterial infections, including sinus or ear infections, and full-blown bronchitis and pneumonia. Some children with slightly narrower or floppier airways may be more susceptible to LTB.

Can you be immune?
Yes, especially if immunized against *H. influenzae* and *S. Pneumoniae*. After you have had a specific viral infection, you are immune to that strain, but each organism has different subtypes, so it is possible to become infected more than once. The *H. influenzae* vaccine has been particularly protective against the high-risk infection called epiglotitis.

What comfort care may be needed?
Gentle nose skin care, extra humidity (this may be particularly helpful), and nasal saline if directed by families. Please note: decongestants and antihistamines (cough and cold medicines) are not helpful and can be potentially harmful for children; they are not recommended.

How can you keep the germs from being spread?
Be sure the child and all care givers have been given appropriate immunizations. Excellent airway hygiene, including aid in covering all coughs and sneezes with disposable tissue, teaching children to

use their sleeves or elbows, and careful hand washing and cleaning of any contaminated surfaces or materials, is necessary to prevent transmission.

How long should the ill child be kept out of child care?
Until fever is gone and the child is comfortable and otherwise doing well, provided the hygiene necessary to control the infection is possible.

What treatments may be needed once the child returns?
No specific treatments may be needed. Follow any treatment plan prescribed by the child's health care provider.

Bronchitis

Bronchitis is an inflammation and infection of the larger airway tubes of the chest. Signs of bronchitis typically include a deep, rough cough, a sore throat, variably hoarse voice, and low-grade fever. It starts as a cold but persists; the cough lasts for more than five days, often longer than twenty days. Children may cough up phlegm or even vomit while coughing because of the amount of mucus in their airway. The usual causes of bronchitis are viral infections of the upper airway, including influenza A and B, parainfluenza, coronavirus (types 1–3), rhinovirus, RSV, and some others. Occasionally bacteria cause bronchitis.

 SPECIAL NOTE about pertussis (whooping cough)

Whooping cough is a serious health problem and is often unrecognized. It takes seven to ten days between exposure and visible illness. Once exposed, a child can spread the germ from seven days after exposure to three weeks after the cough starts, and possibly longer. Whooping cough starts with nonspecific common cold symptoms, including a hacking cough that gradually gets worse. The next stage can last four to twelve weeks and consists of a classic pattern: a series of hard coughs followed by a long, deep intake of breath (the "whoop"), frequently accompanied by vomiting. The coughing slowly improves but can recur with whoop and vomiting for even one to two years. Complications include bronchitis and pneumonia, which can be dangerous especially under age three, and even fatal in infants. Pertussis can be prevented by vaccination. Children are immune after the infection. Adult booster for pertussis is now available.

How is this germ spread?
Germs that cause bronchitis are spread through the airway. They can be directly spread by droplet (through cough or sneeze) or indirectly spread through fresh contamination by an ill person's hands on toys, surfaces, and utensils, including anything that may have been in contact with a contagious child's mouth, nose, or airway secretions, such as straws, silverware, and cups.

How much time elapses between being infected and becoming ill?
Usually twenty-four to forty-eight hours.

When can the child spread the germ?

Bronchitis germs can be spread for several weeks, depending on the germ. A child with whooping cough is contagious for five days after starting medication or twenty-one days from when he starts coughing. Bronchitis caused by influenza and other germs has a highly variable duration of infectiousness.

What are the possible complications?

Progression further into the respiratory tract is not rare and results in bronchiolitis and pneumonia (see pages 21 through 23 for information on these illnesses). Bronchitis frequently causes airway hyperactivity and triggers asthma in susceptible children.

 SPECIAL NOTE about bronchitis

A new infection with bronchitis is importantly different from chronic or recurrent bronchitis. The latter almost always involves some underlying lung problem and needs further evaluation.

Can you be immune?

Vaccination protects against many of these germs, especially *Bordatella pertussis* (whooping cough) and the influenza viruses. Once you have had a specific infection, you can be immune. Because there are many types of most of these germs, it is possible to get new infections.

What comfort care may be needed?

Gentle nose skin care, extra humidity (this may be particularly helpful), and nasal saline if directed by families. Please note: decongestants and antihistamines (cough and cold medicines) are not helpful and can be harmful for children; they are not recommended.

How can you keep the germs from being spread?

Be sure that children and all caregivers have the appropriate immunizations. Excellent airway hygiene, including aid in covering all coughs and sneezes with disposable tissue, teaching children to use their sleeves or elbows, and careful hand washing and cleaning of any contaminated surfaces or materials, is essential to prevent transmission.

How long should the ill child be kept out of child care?

A child with whooping cough must stay out of the child care setting for five days after starting medication or twenty-one days from the start of coughing. Influenza and the other germs may still be spread, but decisions about excluding a child are difficult because the actual germs can rarely be identified. The commonsense recommendation is that a child with bronchitis may return once he no longer has a fever, feels well enough to participate in usual activities, and can cooperate with required hygiene practices, including covering coughs and effective hand washing.

Bronchiolitis

Bronchiolitis is a lower airway tract inflammation or infection of the bronchioles, the next smaller branches of the respiratory tree. The bronchioles bridge between the bronchi and the much smaller alveoli, where the air is exchanged. First symptoms are similar to those of colds, with initial nasal secretion, congestion, and nose tissue swelling. Sneezing, mild sore throat, and low-grade fever may be present. The illness progresses to coughing and more chest symptoms, including more rapid breathing and wheezing. The child's congestion may be so great that she may have trouble sleeping or eating. Bronchiolitis is typically caused by viruses.

How is this germ spread?
Bronchiolitis germs are spread through the airway directly by droplet (through cough or sneeze) or indirectly spread through fresh contamination by an ill person's hands on toys, surfaces, or utensils, including anything that may have been in contact with the contagious child's mouth, nose, or airway secretions, such as straws, silverware, and cups.

How much time elapses between being infected and becoming ill?
Usually around forty-eight hours.

When can the child spread the germ?
For a day before showing signs of illness.

What are the possible complications?
A dangerous risk of apnea (stopping breathing) and respiratory failure exists, particularly among premature infants, low-birth-weight infants, and infants fewer than twelve weeks in age. Children with underlying lung disease, congenital heart disease, immunodeficiency, and defects of the airway are also at increased risk. For the more typical child, complications include pneumonia and secondary bacterial infections of the ears, eyes, and sinuses, as well as triggered asthma.

Can you be immune?
You can be immune to one type of germ, but many germs strains can cause the same illness, so it is possible to become ill again from infections with a different germ type. The highest-risk premature infants can be protected against RSV.

What comfort care may be needed?
Gentle nose skin care, extra humidity, and nasal saline if directed by the child's family. Please note: decongestants and antihistamines (cough and cold medicines) are not helpful and can be harmful for children; they are not recommended.

How can you keep the germs from being spread?
Be sure that children and all caregivers have the appropriate immunizations. Excellent airway hygiene, including aid in covering all coughs and sneezes with disposable tissue, teaching children to use their

sleeves or elbows, and careful hand washing and cleaning of any contaminated surfaces or materials, is crucial to prevent transmission.

How long should the ill child be kept out of child care?

The commonsense recommendation is that the child may return once she is no longer has fever, feels well enough to participate in usual activities, and is able to cooperate with required hygiene practices, including covering coughs and effective hand washing.

Pneumonia

Pneumonia is an inflammation or infection of the lung tissue. Because the infection affects the level of oxygen exchange, a child's ability to get enough oxygen can be affected. This may constitute an emergency. The pattern of pneumonia is not specific and may be very subtle in infants and children. Most children have fever and cough and breathe faster than normal. They may have little appetite and may be restless. Many children also have headaches, pink eyes, a general feeling of being unwell, tiredness, nausea, vomiting accompanying coughing, and stomachaches. Older children may complain of pain with breathing. *Walking pneumonia* is the term used to describe pneumonias with lung symptoms that do not interfere with usual activities.

The germs that can cause pneumonia include viruses, bacteria, and others. They can be, and often are, mixed. Bacterial pneumonia is often caused by *Streptococcus pneumoniae,* which is accompanied by high fever and quick progression of illness to dangerous symptoms of distress. Bacterial infection from mycoplasma or chlamydia can also occur.

How is this germ spread?

These germs can be directly spread by droplet (through cough or sneeze) or indirectly spread through fresh contamination by an ill person's hands on toys, surfaces, and utensils, including anything that may have been in contact with a contagious child's mouth, nose, or airway secretions, such as straws, silverware, and cups.

How much time elapses between being infected and becoming ill?

One to three days or longer, depending on the germ; influenza and *Streptococcus pneumoniae*: one to three days.

When can the child spread the germ?

It depends on the germ. For *Streptococcus pneumoniae,* until twenty-four to forty-eight hours after starting antibiotics. If not treated, the germ can spread for weeks; for influenza, infectiousness lasts at least a week; for most other infection, commonly seven to ten days. Infections such as tuberculosis may remain contagious for years.

What are the possible complications?

Respiratory distress is the greatest danger (see symptoms on page 13). Difficulty feeding can lead to dehydration, which can be especially dangerous in infants. Local complications include lung abscesses, fluid surrounding the lung, and other problems.

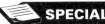 **SPECIAL NOTE about pneumonia**

Recurrent pneumonia is highly associated with underlying lung problems and needs to be evaluated by an appropriate medical provider or specialist.

Can you be immune?

You can be immune to some of the germs. Vaccine protection is available against *Streptococcus pneumoniae* and influenza in particular. Once again, because there are so many strains of the different viruses, you can recover and be immune from one germ and still become sick from a different strain of the germ.

What comfort care may be needed?

Extra humidity is helpful, and nasal saline if directed by families. Please note: decongestants and antihistamines (cough and cold medicines) are not helpful and can be harmful for children; they are not recommended.

How can you keep the germs from being spread?

Be sure the children and all caregivers receive the appropriate immunizations. Excellent airway hygiene, including aid in covering all coughs and sneezes with disposable tissue, teaching children to cover sneezes with their sleeves or elbows, followed by careful hand washing and cleaning of any contaminated surfaces or materials, is essential to prevent transmission.

How long should the ill child be kept out of child care?

The length of time depends on the germ. For *Streptococcus pneumoniae*, the child should remain home at the minimum until twenty-four to forty-eight hours after starting antibiotics. The returning child should be able to feel comfortable, otherwise be doing well, and use the hygiene necessary to control the infection.

Sore Throat

IS THIS AN EMERGENCY?

Call 911 immediately whenever you believe a child has an emergency situation.

Keep the child protected.

Inform the family or guardian as soon as possible.

Refer to the *Medical Emergencies in Early Childhood Settings* Redleaf Quick Guide or another first aid manual as needed.

Because the throat and nose are the entryways for the airway, major problems with them can lead to airway and breathing problems (see the section on airway and breathing problems on page 13). These can constitute emergencies.

Rapidly expanding local infections can cause abscesses and cellulites, which can spread into the bloodstream, spreading infections and causing blood poisoning, sepsis, and shock. Such infections can spread further, causing central nervous system (brain and spinal cord) infections, including meningitis.

What germs can cause this problem?

Most sore throats are caused by either bacterial or viral germs. The most common bacterial problem is strep throat, caused by *Streptococcus pyogenes*, a group A, beta-hemolytic species. Strep throat is unusual because it can cause several complications if not treated with antibiotics. (See below.) Other bacterial germs can cause sore throats, including other species of streptococcus as well as *Staphylococcus aureus.*

Viral germs that cause sore throats include those that cause many common colds, enteroviruses (common summertime viruses that include coxsackie A, which can also cause herpangina and hand, foot, and mouth disease), and Epstein-Barr (mononucleosis).

What is the likely pattern of this illness?

A child infected by these germs shows a pattern that moves quickly from starting to feel ill to significant discomfort within hours. Fever and reluctance to eat or drink are common. Toddlers often have runny noses as well as sore throats. Older children often have upset stomach as well.

Each of the following illnesses can cause sore throat symptoms and can follow slightly different patterns.

- **Strep throat:** Strep throat is very rare in babies under one year. It can cause a very sore throat that appears very raw and red across the back of the throat, including the soft palate and tonsils.

Sometimes it causes swollen glands under the jaw. Some strains can cause scarlatina, a condition in which a sandpapery, fine red rash spreads over the chest and trunk. A more severe form of strep illness called *scarlet fever* includes scarlatina body rash, a red, tender tongue, and eventual peeling of the fingertips and toes.

- **Mononucleosis:** Commonly called *mono*, this infection usually causes extreme tiredness and may well include other symptoms, such as rash, achiness, and malaise.

- **Influenza:** Influenza, or the flu (described in the section on upper respiratory infections beginning on page 16), can cause a very sore throat following the initial, sudden symptoms of fever, chills, headache, muscle aches, and cough.

- **Enterovirus infections:** Enteroviral infections most commonly cause sore throats with mouth sores, fever, and some cold symptoms. Children with these infections can also develop rashes. Hand, foot, and mouth disease (Coxsackie A virus) is one version with fever and sores on the inside of the lips, mouth, and tongue, especially toward the front of the mouth. Coxsackie also can cause a rash with small, oval, tender, flat sores on the palms of the hands, soles of the feet, and, less commonly, the buttocks.

- **Herpangina:** Herpangina can be caused by Coxsackie A virus. This infection causes fever and very sore throat, with tender, blistered mouth sores, usually on the tonsils and soft palate.

How is this germ spread?

These germs can be directly spread by droplet (through cough or sneeze). Some germs (including the summertime enterovirus) are spread by fecal and oral routes. Both kinds can be indirectly spread through fresh contamination by an ill person's hands on toys, surfaces, and utensils, including anything that may have been in contact with a contagious child's mouth, nose, or airway secretions, such as straws, silverware, and cups.

How much time elapses between being infected and becoming ill?

Strep throat: two to five days; mono: thirty to fifty days; influenza: about fourteen days; enterovirus infection: three to six days.

When can the child spread the germ?

For strep throat, a child is often contagious for one day before she shows any signs of illness until twenty-four hours after starting appropriate antibiotics. Viral infections vary but can be contagious before the child exhibits any symptoms.

What are the possible complications?

Strep throat has a couple of unusual complications, including abscesses near and around the tonsil called *peritonsillar* (formerly called *quinsy*) or *retropharyngeal* or *lymph node abscesses*. All of these need immediate care. Untreated strep is the germ most likely to cause acute rheumatic fever with joint pain, ongoing fevers, and rash. This condition can ultimately cause chorea (brain problems) and carditis (heart problems and value problems with heart failure). Untreated strep throat can cause post infectious acute renal failure, a form of kidney failure called *acute glomerulonephritis*. (Other illnesses may also cause this kidney problem, but strep throat is overwhelmingly the most common cause.) Very rarely, strep throat can cause arthritis (joint infection). Other complications of strep include ear and sinus infections.

Can you be immune?

You cannot be immune to strep throat. Once you have been infected by specific strains, you are unlikely to contract the same illness again. But most bacterial infections are caused by many different strains, and it is possible to become infected by slightly different ones.

Once you have had mono, you are not susceptible to reinfection, and the original infection can rarely be reactivated.

What comfort care may be needed?

Keep the child comfortable, using fluids and fever and pain control as instructed by the family or health provider until the family takes the child home.

How can you keep the germs from being spread?

Once you have identified an ill child, keep her away from close contact with other children.

How long should the ill child be kept out of child care?

For strep, the child should remain at home for twenty-four hours after starting appropriate antibiotics. For viral sore throats, deciding when the child can return is more difficult because she can still share the virus for several weeks or longer. The best advice is to have the child stay home until her fever is gone and she is eating and drinking normally.

What treatments may be needed once the child returns?

The child should be able to return to all activities once she returns. If she had strep and is still on antibiotics, you will need to continue the medication on the schedule set up by her medical provider.

Abdominal and Digestive Problems

IS THIS AN EMERGENCY?

Call 911 immediately if you ever believe the child has an emergency situation.

Keep the child protected.

Inform the family or guardian as soon as possible.

Refer to the *Medical Emergencies in Early Childhood Settings* Redleaf Quick Guide or another first aid manual as needed.

Two main kinds of emergencies arise from problems in the abdomen and digestive organs. The first is structural: organs within the abdomen can present surgical problems, such as when the intestines become twisted (malrotation), blocked (obstruction), telescoped (intussusception), or infected (appendicitis). These are rare conditions sometimes associated with infection. The second kind of emergency is functional: it can include vomiting or diarrhea, which may lead to severe dehydration, shock, or chemical imbalances that can lead to seizures, muscle spasms, and more. These symptoms are frequently caused by infections and can be highly contagious.

Babies and toddlers are at high risk for vomiting and diarrhea and other food and waterborne illness because of frequent hand-to-mouth contact and limited preexisting immunity. Babies and toddlers can become dehydrated much more quickly than adults.

What germs can cause this problem?

Viruses, such as rotavirus, bacteria, such as E. Coli, and parasites, such as giardia, can cause these infections.

Germs can infect the liver, causing hepatitis. Almost always viral, the most common ones are hepatitis A, hepatitis B, hepatitis C, and cytomegalovirus.

What is the likely pattern of this illness?

Two pathways cause the vomiting and/or diarrhea: either direct invasion of the wall of the abdomen or production of an enterotoxin that chemically causes the symptoms. Germs can cause faster movement of food through the digestive system (hypermotility), which produces diarrhea by decreasing the time that is needed for normal absorption of food and fluids. They can also slow movement, producing impaired peristasis or ileus when completely stopped, thereby causing inflammation. If they increase in number rapidly, they may keep nutrients from being absorbed into the body (malabsorption).

Hepatitis triggers many problems because the liver is a major factory of many things the body needs. The classic pattern includes a general feeling of illness, lack of appetite, nausea, jaundice (yellowing of the skin, especially the whites of the eyes), and sometimes abdominal pain, fever, diarrhea, fatigue, and/or itching.

How is this germ spread?

Rotavirus, the most common abdominal infection among children six to twenty-four months, seems most infectious in autumn and winter and is transmitted from stool to mouth as well as through the air. Calicivirses are around all year and are transmitted from stool to mouth and through water, can be found in contaminated food, including shellfish, and may also be airborne. Astrovirus are found in winter and are transmitted stool to mouth. Enteric adenoviruses are summertime viruses and are spread the same way.

Salmonella, campylobacter, *Escherichia coli*, shigella, and *Staphylococcus aureus* are spread through contaminated food. Cryptosporidium is waterborne. Clostridium's (botulism) spore toxin is rare but potentially life-threatening and is spread in contaminated food. Most people have symptoms from ingesting already-produced toxin. Infants can ingest the spores and then incubate the germ, which then makes and releases the toxin.

Hepatitis A is spread from stool to mouth as well as through contaminated water or food. Hepatitis B, hepatitis C, and cytomegalovirus (CMV) can be transmitted before and around birth but can also be spread later through blood contamination (including blood products and even dried blood). CMV can also be spread through the airway and saliva and even through urine.

How much time elapses between being infected and becoming ill?

As little as an hour if a person eats food contaminated with toxin (food poisoning) or up to several days or weeks for some of the other infections that cause vomiting and diarrhea. Hepatitis B can take one to four months. It takes fifteen to fifty days to become sick from hepatitis A. Hepatitis C may take years, and little else about its incubation period is known. Cytomegalovirus can be days to months.

When can the child spread the germ?

From the onset of vomiting or diarrhea until no loose stool has occurred for twenty-four hours. Some germs continue to be shed through bowel movements for weeks to months. For the hepatitis viruses, a child can typically spread the germs for weeks to months; many children may shed them for years.

What are the possible complications?

Complications are related to water and salt loss. Severe dehydration can lead to shock. Brain injury and nerve injury can occur because of changes in salt levels. Death can occur if a child is not rehydrated quickly and appropriately.

Complications from hepatitis include liver failure, development of chronic hepatitis, and (rarely) liver cancer (hepatitis B).

Can you be immune?

You can be immunized to rotavirus, hepatitis A, and hepatitis B. Otherwise, you are at risk for each new strain of the germs that cause these many abdominal infections. A rotavirus vaccine is available, but it must be started within the first two months of life and follow a specific schedule.

What comfort care may be needed?

Keep the child comfortable and well hydrated. Pain management should be directed by the family and/or the child's medical provider. Please note: antivomiting and antidiarrhea medications are rarely helpful and can be harmful for children; they are never recommended unless specifically directed by the family and medical provider.

How can you keep the germs from being spread?

Isolate the ill child and arrange for him to go home as soon as possible. Maintain effective hand-washing technique and general cleaning of potentially contaminated surfaces and materials. Diapers and pull-ups should be placed in tightly closed bags and taken directly outside to the trash. Hand washing before and after diaper and toilet assistance for both staff and children is recommended. Cleaning the diaper changing area after use is always recommended.

How long should the ill child be kept out of child care?

The commonsense plan is until twenty-four hours after the child's last loose stool or vomiting ends.

Inflamed Eyes

IS THIS AN EMERGENCY?

Call 911 immediately if you ever believe the child has an emergency situation.

Keep the child protected.

Inform the family or guardian as soon as possible.

Refer to the *Medical Emergencies in Early Childhood Settings* Redleaf Quick Guide or another first aid manual as needed.

There are very few infection conditions that can be emergencies, but rapidly swelling, red eyelids and tissue around the eyes (periorbital cellulitis) or any concern about vision or eye pain including pain with light (photophobia), especially with severe headache and nausea, can be dangerous and needs immediate evaluation.

What germs can cause this problem?

Infectious conjunctivitis is typically caused by bacterial germs *(Staphylococcus aureus, Streptococcus pneumoniae, Haemophilus influenzae, Moraxella catarrhalis*, and *chlamydia)* or viral infections (adenovirus in particular).

What is the likely pattern of this illness?

Pink eye is a term that has come to mean any concern about the eyes, including tearing, matting, crusting, or other eyelid pinkness or redness. True pink eye is called *conjunctivitis*, which means irritation of the lining of the white part of the eye. All children with conjunctivitis have red eyes, but not all children with red eyes have conjunctivitis. All children with red eyes need evaluation. Acute conjunctivitis is often caused by factors other than germs, such as allergies and other kinds of inflammation, including chemical irritation. As for the classic infection, one or both eyes may be red, with tearing (especially from viruses) or matting (white, yellow, or green—the latter especially in cases of bacterial infections). Sometimes eyes may become "stuck shut," especially after sleeping.

How is this germ spread?

It is spread by direct contact with secretions or contaminated objects and surfaces.

How much time elapses between being infected and becoming ill?

As few as twelve hours.

When can the child spread the germ?

The germ can be spread as soon as the child has symptoms.

What are the possible complications?

The infection can spread into the tissues around the eye and backward into the eye (orbital cellulitis) and the brain (causing abscess, meningitis, or encephalitis).

Can you be immune?

There are vaccines for *Hemophilus influenzae* and *Streptococcus pneumoniae*. Each bacterium has many subgroups, and it is possible for them to have many strains. Recurrent or persistent pink eye may be a sign of other eye problems and should be evaluated.

What comfort care may be needed?

Gentle skin care and warm compresses, if directed by the family.

How can you keep the germs from being spread?

Children should not share tissues, towels, linens, or silverware. Effective hand washing is always recommended.

How long should the ill child be kept out of child care?

Bacterial conjunctivitis is contagious until treated for twenty-four hours. There is no need to keep children away with nonbacterial causes of conjunctivitis.

Joint Problems

What germs can cause this problem?

Bacterial infections with *Hemophilus influenzae*, *Staphylococcus aureus*, Group B streptococcus, and *Escherichia coli* are the most common. *Mycobacterium tuberculosis* and rare fungi, including *Coccidioides immitis*, can cause joint infections. Lyme disease, caused by a tick-born infection with the spirochete *Borrelia burgdorferi*, can produce longer-term symptoms of joint problems with intermittent or persistent pain and swelling in one or more large joints.

What is the likely pattern of this illness?

It is never normal for a child to have abnormal joints. Joint infection is rarely the issue; usually joint problems are the result of injury or systemic illnesses that are not infections. All joint concerns need to be evaluated. Children with joint infections may have fevers and rashes, in addition to red, swollen, painful joints. They may have functional changes, including limps or decreased normal use. Infections can be local (septic arthritis) or can involve multiple joints (as in Lyme disease or after infection with strep, parvovirus, and others).

How is this germ spread?

Usually from infections present in a child's upper airway, nose, ears, or mouth, or from skin entry sites, then moving through the child's blood stream.

How much time elapses between being infected and becoming ill?

It can be as few as several hours, depending on the germ.

When can the child spread the germ?

The germs that cause joint infections do not spread to other children directly.

What are the possible complications?

Local damage may include arthritis. The infection may also spread throughout the body, including the blood, leading to shock and sepsis.

Can you be immune?

There is no immunity for this type of germ.

What comfort care may be needed?

Gentle care and support of the sore joint, including allowing the child to rest as needed.

How can you keep the germs from being spread?

Follow the same care you would for all upper airway and respiratory illnesses.

How long should the ill child be kept out of child care?

If the joint problem was caused by germs, the child should not return to child care until his infection is mostly resolved and his activity level is almost back to normal.

What treatments may be needed once the child returns?

Follow the family's directions and any treatment plan from the child's medical provider.

Rashes and Other Skin or Scalp Changes

IS THIS AN EMERGENCY?

Call 911 immediately if you ever believe the child has an emergency situation.

Keep the child protected.

Inform the family or guardian as soon as possible.

Refer to the *Medical Emergencies in Early Childhood Settings* Redleaf Quick Guide or another first aid manual as needed.

What germs can cause this problem?

Bacteria including *Staphylococcus aureus* and Group A streptococcus, among others, can cause impetigo with crusty or red skin. Bacteria can also cause deeper abscesses (boils).

Viruses, including those that cause measles, mumps, chicken pox, rubella (German measles), hand, foot, and mouth disease, cold sores, roseola, and fifth disease cause classic childhood rashes. There are many other viruses that can have associated rashes.

What is the likely pattern of the illness?

Each of the following viruses can produce vague symptoms, including fever, fussiness, and runny nose. Each has its own pattern of rash. (Remember: it is not up to you to diagnosis a specific illness but to alert the family, comfort the child, and protect the other children from likely risk.)

1. **Measles** takes ten to twelve days between infection and visible illness. The child remains contagious from the fifth day after infection until several days after the rash appears. The child experiences congestion, cough, pink eyes, and fever for three to four days before the rash. She is most likely to be contagious just before the rash appears. Complications can include pneumonia, ear infections, airway laryngitis (which may be an emergency) and brain infections (these can be deadly). Measles can be prevented by vaccination. After the illness is over, the child is immune from measles.

2. **Rubella (German measles)** takes fourteen to twenty-one days between infection and visible illness. The maximum time a child can infect others is from seven days before to five days after the rash appears. The first symptom is the rash, but the child may have low-grade fever, headache, pink eyes, sore throat, and cough. Many enlarged lymph nodes may accompany the rash. Complications are rare, but a child may develop arthritis from rubella. The biggest danger is spreading the infection to a pregnant, nonimmune woman, which can cause problems for her unborn child. Rubella can be prevented by vaccination. After the illness is over, the child is immune from rubella.

3. **Roseola** takes nine to fifteen days from infection to visible illness. An infected child is contagious from shortly before he gets the fever until the fever breaks. The classic infection has high and continuous fever for three to four days; a rash appears when the fever breaks. The primary complication is febrile seizures, which are rare. After the illness is over, the child is immune from roseola.

4. **Chicken pox (varicella)** takes ten to twenty-one days from infection to visible illness. The child is contagious from one day before any showing any signs of being ill until all pox have crusted. The child often has a low-grade fever and generally doesn't feel well. Complications include secondary infections of the crusts by other germs and possible spread of these infections through the blood (see the section on shock on page 9), brain infection, and pneumonia. Chicken pox can be prevented by vaccination. After the illness is over, the child is immune from chicken pox.

5. **Mumps** takes sixteen to eighteen days from infection to physical illness. A child can spread the infection from the start of illness until nine days after swelling became visible. The illness starts with fever, headache, and a general feeling of being unwell. A child sometime complains of pain on the side of the face, which then progresses to swelling and tenderness to one or both parotid salivary glands (parotitis), although symptoms vary. Mumps may include testicular infection (epididymo-orchitis) and brain infections. Complications may include partial atrophy of the male testicles. Mumps can be prevented by vaccination. After the illness, the child is immune from mumps.

6. **Parvovirus B19** can cause fifth disease, an infection causing mild fever and classic rash with a slapped-face appearance and a body rash (erythema infectiosum). The infected child may have joint pain, especially later. Children with underlying blood problems (hemolytic disorders) may develop bone marrow failure. The biggest danger is spreading the infection to a pregnant, nonimmune woman, which can lead to the death of her fetus. After the illness is over, the child is immune from parvovirus.

In addition to viral infections, rashes can be caused by bacteria and fungi. The following are among the most common.

1. **Lyme disease** has several phases, with a possible initial skin "target" lesion, which may be followed weeks later by skin rashes, along with heart and brain or nerve problems, and later still by joint and other brain problems. It is caused by bacteria introduced through a tick bite. It is not contagious.

2. **Monilia** is an infection with *Candida albicans*. It may be oral (thrush, with white patches in the mouth) and on the skin (diaper rashes, with red, raw areas that can spread and be itchy and painful). It rarely has complications. It is spread through saliva and from stool to mouth. Maintain excellent hygiene, including hand washing before and after diapering or toileting, and clean any material that has come in contact with saliva. Thrush will need medical evaluation.

3. **Tinea or ringworm** is caused by several species of fungi. They may infect the body (*Tinea corporis* on trunk and limbs), the head and scalp (*Tinea capitis*), or the groin (*Tinea cruris*). An infected child may experience itching and patches of skin with central clearing, variable hair loss, and occasionally a larger, thick boggy patch called a *kerion*. All of these problems require medical evaluation. Effective hand washing and avoidance of direct skin-to-skin contamination are the best way to prevent transmission.

Warts

Warts are common problems for children, but they are not highly contagious. Children with warts should not need to be excluded from child care. *Molluscum contagiosum* warts can be anywhere on the body, including the face. The disease may be itchy and presents as smooth bumps with a dimpled surface. The warts don't become red unless irritated. Plantar warts are on the soles of the feet and palms of the hand and are usually small areas with slightly hardened, thickened skin.

Urinary Tract Infections

What germs can cause this problem?

Escherichia coli bacteria are the most common pathogens and cause the infection about 80 percent of the time. Other bacteria include stool germs of the genuses *klebsiella, proteus, enterobacter, citrobacter, enterococcus*, and the species *Staphylococcus saprophyticus* and *Staphylococcus aureus*. Viruses include adenovirus, enterovirus, coxsackievirus, and echovirus. Fungi that cause infections include candida, cryptococcus, and aspergillus species, but usually only children with immune problems or those who have used antibiotics for extended periods are susceptible.

What is the likely pattern of this illness?

Urinary tract infections are extremely subtle and therefore are often missed. Sometimes the only symptom you can observe is fever, especially in infants. Sometimes the urine seems changed—the odor, color, or child's normal pattern of urination changes. Be sure to share any concern about the child's urine pattern with her family. Classic symptoms of UTI include painful urination, urgency (a strong need to go), urinating more or less frequently, and fever.

Lower tract infections often cause misery with painful urination, abdomen pain, nausea, incontinence (wetting), vomiting, fevers (often extremely high), chills, urgent and frequent need to urinate, and more. Upper tract infections can share these signs and are more likely to include back or flank pain. Girls are affected much more commonly than boys.

How is this germ spread?

In newborns, UTIs are most commonly spread by blood infections (bacteremia). Once a child is slightly older, infection enters the bladder from the skin of the groin or a caregiver's infected hand. This type of infection is called an *ascending infection.*

How much time elapses between being infected and becoming ill?

Illness or symptoms may appear within hours.

When can the child spread the germ?

Because all the germs are standard stool germs, the germ can be spread during diapering or toileting. (Excellent individual hygiene and diaper and toilet hygiene must be routine practice.)

What are the possible complications?

Upper tract infections (pyelonephritis) may lead to kidney scars, high blood pressure, and kidney failure.

Can you be immune?

No.

What comfort care may be needed?

Gentle, normal skin care for the groin area.

How can you keep the germs from being spread?

This is primarily an individual vulnerability, but excellent hygiene, such as wiping girls from front to back in the diapering and toilet areas is vital. This includes proper hand-washing technique both before and after diapering or toileting.

How long should the ill child be kept out of child care?

This depends on the child's comfort level. When the child can participate fully in activities, she can return.

What treatments may be needed once the child returns?

If treatment is needed, follow the treatment plan supplied by the child's family or medical provider.

Ear Infections

What germs can cause this problem?

The bacteria that most typically cause ear infections include *Streptococcus pneumoniae*, *Haemophilus influenzae*, and *Moxacella catarrhalis*. Viral infections with respiratory syncytial viruses, *coronavirus*, rhinovirus, and influenza A and B are possible. Other pathogens, rare but possible, include *Mycoplasma pneumoniae*, *Chlamydohila pneumoniae*, and *Mycobacterium tuberculosis*.

What is the likely pattern of this illness?

Ear infections (otitis media) swell the middle ear with fluid, causing pain. Sometimes the child exhibits decreased appetite, restless sleeping, fever, and decreased hearing.

How is this germ spread?

Ear infections are not directly contagious. Generally, ear infections are secondary to upper respiratory infections or common colds. While ear infections are not contagious, upper respiratory infections are. (See the section on upper respiratory infections beginning on page 16.) Always feeding infants with their heads elevated may decrease the rate of ear infections.

How much time elapses between being infected and becoming ill?

Typically several days from common cold with congestion until fluid develops in the middle ear.

When can the child spread the germ?

Ear infections are not contagious. The common cold can be spread. (See the section on upper respiratory infections beginning on page 16.)

What are the possible complications?

If the fluid does not clear from the middle ear, persistent hearing loss may occur, leading to problems in language and speech and impaired general development. Ear drum perforation, local spread with mastoiditis and sinus infections, meningitis (infection of the brain covering), brain abscesses, and blood vessel infections with clotting may be serious complications.

Can you be immune?

Vaccination for *Streptococcus pneumoniae* is protective. Once you have had a specific infection, you may be immune. But again, since there are many strains of most of these germs, it is possible to get new infections. Avoiding pacifier use and smoke are preventive measures.

What comfort care may be needed?

Pain management should be directed by the family. Please note: decongestants and antihistamines (cough and cold medicines) are not helpful and can be harmful for children; they are not recommended.

How can you keep the germs from being spread?

Excellent airway hygiene, including aid in covering all coughs and sneezes with disposable tissue, teaching children to cover sneezes with their sleeves or elbows, and careful hand washing and cleaning of any contaminated surfaces or materials, is necessary to prevent transmission.

How long should the ill child be kept out of child care?

By the time most children develop an ear infection, the cold is passing or has passed. At that point, they should not be considered infectious and do not need to be restricted from child care, provided their comfort level and ability to handle normal activities are good.

Part 3: Immunizations

Immunizations are the most effective way to prevent certain infections. They allow a person to develop a protective immune response without the risk of actual infection. Immunization protects the individual and others by avoiding further spread of the disease. This conferred protection includes others too young to be immunized, people who were vaccinated but did not mount a good immune response, and people who have chosen for either medical or personal reasons not to be immunized.

It is important that all child care providers and children receive all of the vaccinations recommended for their age. Because you are responsible for the young children in your care, it is especially important that you are immune to vaccine-preventable childhood diseases to protect yourself *and* to prevent infection of children who may not be fully immune. All staff and children should provide a copy of their immunization records to the child care site. Those children and staff members who are not immunized should be considered for exclusion from child care during outbreaks of certain infectious diseases (whooping cough, for example) even if they seem healthy.

Child care providers should have either proven immunity or up-to-date immunization for

- diphtheria, tetanus, and pertussis (whooping cough);

- hepatitis A;

- hepatitis B;

- influenza (flu);

- measles, mumps, and rubella (German measles);

- varicella (chicken pox).

Speak with your medical provider about your need for vaccination. First of all, make sure your provider understands your occupation—that you work with infants and young children. Clarify your vaccination history, review possible contraindications and precautions, and see if you need to be tested for existing antibody or immune status. Then determine exactly how best to get the vaccines you need.

The nationally recommended Adult Immunization Schedule from the Centers for Disease Control and Prevention (CDC) is available on the CDC Web site in English and Spanish: www.cdc.gov/vaccines/recs/schedules/adult-schedule.htm.

General information about adult vaccinations is available from state and local health departments and from CDC at www.cdc.gov/vaccines. Vaccine information statements are available at www.cdc.gov/vaccines/pubs/vis. You can view, download, and print Advisory Committee on Immunization Practices (ACIP) statements for each recommended vaccine and provisional vaccine recommendations at www.cdc.gov/vaccines/pubs/acip-list.htm.

State-by-state mandates for children in child care can be found several places, including www.cdc.gov/vaccines/recs/schedules/child-schedule.htm and www.immunize.org/laws. These schedules indicate the recommended ages for routine administration of currently licensed childhood vaccines.

They are updated on the Web sites, so the most current versions can be found online. The Recommended Immunization Schedules for Persons Aged 0–18 Years are approved by the Advisory Committee on Immunization Practices at www.cdc.gov/vaccines/recs/acip, the American Academy of Pediatrics, www.aap.org, and the American Academy of Family Physicians, www.aafp.org. All of these sites have helpful information for families.

 SPECIAL NOTE about family immunizations

Effective immunizations have helped reduce or eliminate many infectious diseases and are responsible for preventing millions of illnesses and deaths in children every year. The benefit of immunization extends beyond the immunized individual and is a true public health benefit. Despite the success of immunizations, some families refuse to immunize their children. They have many reasons for doing so, including concerns about the pain of the process, religious or philosophical convictions, and the belief that the benefits of vaccinations do not justify the risks. Vaccines are very safe, but they are not risk free. Nor are they 100 percent effective. Almost everything in a child's world has risks and benefits—their food, medicine, and personal experiences for growth and development. Decisions about vaccination affect children and the people who are in their immediate world. The families of the children in your care should be directed to their medical providers to discuss the matter. The welfare of their children needs to be the primary focus for families. Your focus must be on deciding what is in the best interests of you, your staff, and the other children in your care. For the most up-to-date information about vaccines and immunizations, check the following Web sites:

- American Academy of Pediatrics (AAP) • www.aap.org

- Childhood Immunization Support Program • www.cispimmunize.org

- Every Child by Two • www.ecbt.org

- Immunization Action Coalition • www.immunize.org

- National Immunization Program • www.cdc.gov/vaccines

- National Network for Immunization Information • www.immunizationinfo.org

Part 4: Breaking the Chain of Infection

There are many ways to help break the chain of infection and provide a healthier environment for yourself, your staff, and the children in your care.

- Compile illness and immunization records for children and child care providers.

- Train and reinforce proper hand-washing technique.

- Improve personal hygiene for both children and child care providers.

- Enforce sanitary food preparation and handling.

- Clean and sanitize your site.

Compile Illness and Immunization Records for Children and Child Care Providers

It is extremely helpful for both you and the families of the children in your care to have clear policies and simple ways to record health issues, including ongoing medical illnesses or problems, allergies, medications, and immunizations.

Your initial registration or enrollment form for each child needs to contain a section for medical information, including

- All appropriate contact information as well as the best method of contact

- Who should be notified in case of an emergency or illness, with home, work, and mobile phone numbers

- Who is authorized to pick up the child in case of illness

- Who the preferred medical provider (or medical group) is, with phone numbers

- Which hospital is preferred, with phone number

- Medications

- Allergies

- Medical diagnosis or conditions (for example, skin conditions, frequent ear problems, asthma)

- Any special instructions needed

- Complete and up-to-date immunization history

- Weight and height (up-to-date)

A child care log form is useful for daily reporting of accidents, illnesses, unusual behavior, and other observations. Families need information from you to understand their child and their child's world.

Train and Reinforce Proper Hand-Washing Technique

Hand washing with soap and water can be taught and needs to be done well. Proper hand washing needs to be consistent and supervised until it becomes a habit! Liquid soap, running water, and enough time are the three key elements.

Rinse first with water, then count to ten as you vigorously lather the entire hand, including between the fingers, under the fingernails, and all around the wrists, with liquid soap. Many children too young to count can learn to sing a song that lasts long enough for a proper wash. After soaping, rinse off under the running water for as long as it takes to count to ten. Turn off the tap with a paper towel and use a new towel to pat the hands dry. Carefully dispose of used towels.

The soap should make bubbles easily and should be tolerated by the staff and children. It does not have to be a harsh, antigerm formula. Liquid soap is preferable to bar soap because soap bars can actually grow germs. It is important to not recontaminate hands on the faucet or the soap container, which is why you should use a disposable paper towel to turn off the faucet when the hand washing is complete.

Because cracks in the skin may be uncomfortable as well as provide an avenue for germs to enter the body, be sure to use moisturizers. Proper technique should be used to avoid transmission here too.

> Hand washing is the single most important way to control and prevent the spread of germs.

LIMIT USE OF ALCOHOL SANITIZERS

It is always preferable to use soap and water if there is a choice. Alcohol sanitizers are better than nothing if either you or a child has been contaminated and you cannot get to soap and water in a reasonable amount of time. Alcohol can be very harsh on the skin, often causing irritation and cracking, especially in young children. Most important, alcohol sanitizers kill only some of the germs. In contrast, soap and water lift and float off all kinds of germs.

Improve Personal Hygiene for Both Children and Child Care Providers

Several personal hygiene issues affect children and the adults who care for them.

- Proper times for hand washing

- Covering coughs and sneezes

- Proper diapering and toileting

PROPER TIMES TO WASH YOUR OWN HANDS

It is always appropriate for adults to wash their hands, and your staff need to be encouraged to wash their hands often. In particular, they should always wash their hands

- when arriving at the child care setting (before the children arrive);

- before and after handling food;

- after touching pets;

- before and after eating;

- before and after changing a child's diaper or assisting in his toilet care;

- before and after using the toilet themselves;

- after touching their own or a child's face, including aid in wiping a nose;

- before and after cleaning up a child's body fluid, including saliva, vomit, urine, or stool;

- after taking out or handling trash or garbage;

- before leaving the child care setting (or after the children have left).

PROPER TIMES FOR CHILDREN TO WASH THEIR HANDS

It is always appropriate to help children wash their hands or supervise older children's hand washing. Proper hand washing for children needs to be encouraged, reinforced, and, most of all, modeled by adults. Children should wash their hands (or have their hands washed)

- when they first arrive;

- before and after eating;

- after touching pets;

- after coughing or sneezing;

- if they touch another child's face or body fluids;

- before and after a diaper change or toileting;

- before and after going outside;

- just before they go home.

COVERING COUGHS AND SNEEZES

Airborne particles are hard to stop, but properly covering coughs and sneezes certainly helps. Teach children to cover a cough or sneeze by coughing or sneezing into their upper sleeves, inside their elbow area, or into a tissue. They should be taught not to use their hands. Children should wash their hands properly after coughing or sneezing.

DIAPER AND TOILET CARE

A specific area must be set aside for diaper changes. Do not set up a diapering area near areas where food is prepared, stored, or eaten. All supplies need to be ready and easily available. Enough space should be provided, and you should clean the area after every use and then wash your hands. Consider using a roll of paper, such as the kind doctors use on examining tables, that can cover the changing pad and then be torn off and disposed of after each use. Be sure to dispose of dirty diapers and wipes, including toilet paper, without contaminating other areas.

While many centers use gloves (non-latex), good hygiene is possible without them. Use proper hand-washing technique for both yourself and the child before and after, whether gloves are used or not.

For older children who toilet themselves with little or no adult help, make sure they properly wash their hands before and after toileting. Check and clean the toilet area as needed after children have finished. Properly dispose of paper towels, toilet paper, and other soiled paper.

Enforce Sanitary Food Preparation and Handling

Your state and local health departments and licensing authority provide you with guidelines for food storage, preparation, and cooking. These guidelines were created to help prevent illnesses that can be caused by foods contaminated by germs. It is important for you and your staff to review those guidelines regularly and to follow them closely. Most are commonsense guidlines. Following these guidelines can greatly reduce the risk of introducing food-borne illnesses into your early childhood setting. Remember to

- wash hands and surfaces properly and frequently;

- refrigerate all foods properly;

- avoid cross contamination by keeping foods separate;

- follow health department guidelines for proper preparation and cooking.

Clean and Sanitize Your Site

You need to provide a clean and safe place for your staff and the children in your care. All cleaning products that you're using must be safe to be used around children of all ages. All cleaning supplies must be locked away safely so that children can't get to them.

DISINFECTING

Disinfection kills almost all bacteria, fungi, viruses, and parasites. It reduces the number of micro-organisms, making equipment and surfaces safer for use. Bleach solution remains the gold standard for cleaning and disinfecting bathrooms, diaper areas, kitchen, tables, and appropriately textured toys and other materials.

Normally, ordinary household bleach has a 5.0 percent chlorine concentration. The Centers for Disease Control recommends preparing two solutions (stronger and weaker) of ordinary household bleach. Bleach solutions must be prepared daily and clearly labeled with the correct concentration. They lose their strength after twenty-four hours. Any time the odor of chlorine is not present, discard the solution. When preparing these solutions, be sure to use proper ventilation.

Strong Solution

A strong bleach-to-water solution with a ratio of 1 to 10 can be used to disinfect areas that are likely to be contaminated with stool (bathrooms, changing areas) or other body fluids, including blood, vomit, or other emissions from an infected child.

Weaker Solution

A weaker bleach-to-water solution with a ratio of 1 to 100 is used to disinfect hard surfaces and toys. To make this concentration, use one part of the stronger 1 to 10 solution and then add 9 equal parts of water.

 SPECIAL NOTE about using bleach solutions

The strong bleach solution is caustic. Avoid direct contact with skin and eyes. Both the strong and weaker solutions can bleach clothing if splashed or not given proper time to dry. Have plenty of paper towels available to wipe the area nearly dry, or allow at least a three-minute drying period before touching.

Resources for Providers and Families

Health Organizations

American Academy of Family Physicians • www.aafp.org and www.familydoctor.org

American Academy of Pediatrics • www.aap.org

American Academy of Pediatrics Childhood Immunization Support Program • www.cispimmunize.org

American Nurses Association • www.nursingworld.org

Association for Prevention Teaching and Research • www.aptrweb.org

UpToDate for Patients • www.uptodate.com/patients

Nonprofit Groups and Universities

All Kids Count • www.allkidscount.org

Every Child by Two • www.ecbt.org

Immunization Action Coalition • www.immunize.org

Institute for Vaccine Safety at Johns Hopkins Bloomberg School of Public Health • www.vaccine safety.edu

National Foundation for Infectious Diseases • www.nfid.org

National Network for Immunization Information • www.immunizationinfo.org

National Association for the Education of Young Children • www.naeyc.org

Government

Centers for Disease Control and Prevention (CDC) • www.cdc.gov

National Association of County and City Health Officials • www.naccho.org

Index of Common Illnesses